Reach for the Dream!

Developing Individual Service Plans for Persons with Disabilities

Second Edition

By Dale DiLeo

**Development supported by:
The New Hampshire Division
of Mental Health and
Developmental Services**

TRN Training Resource Network ✦ St. Augustine, Florida

Printed in the United States of America by Rose Printing

Published by Training Resource Network (TRN), PO Box 439, St. Augustine, FL 32085-0439. You may order prepaid directly from the publisher for $20.00 plus $3.00 shipping and handling per copy. Florida orders please add state sales tax.

ISBN 1-883302-01-3
Second Edition

Contents

Introduction

In recent years, there has been a growing recognition of the need for more effective life planning for people with disabilities. While each state requires some sort of written plan of funded services, many of these plans are inadequate in addressing the real life needs of the person at the center of them.

In New Hampshire, a group of people called "case managers" was given the task of facilitating individual service plans (ISPs) for persons with disabilities. These individuals, with the support of the Division of Mental Health and Developmental Services, also felt the need to revise the planning process used to better reflect more personalized life enhancement principles.

Over the course of a year and a half, through demanding retreats and trainings, a consensus emerged about values, processes, and strategies for individual service planning for the future. I was pleased to act as the facilitator for many of these sessions in which people challenged old structures and each other to try to build a better service support system.

Reach for the Dream! is a reflection of that consensus. This second edition includes updated information on person-centered planning. This is based on both my own personal experiences and the work of many other people involved in helping people plan better lives.

Because of the need for individual flexibility, there is no fixed checklist of procedures contained here. Since constantly evolving standards in every state and province do have certain requirements for the planning process and the finished document, the people who facilitate planning meetings should carefully review the regulations and standards that govern them.

Many persons provided input and advice during the course of this endeavor. Thanks should particularly be given to *Mike Shields*, Training Director at the New Hampshire Division of Mental Health and Developmental Services; *Robert Vaillancourt*, Case Management Supervisor for United Developmental Services in Lebanon, NH; *Dawn Langton*, Director of DL Networks in St. Augustine, FL; and *Debra Nelson*, Project Director at the Institute on Disability/University of New Hampshire, for their support, guidance, and editorial assistance.

Thanks also to all the individuals and their families and friends who agree to work with facilitators and professionals in partnership for life planning. Finally, thank you to all those who work in community support services for persons with disabilities in New Hampshire, the first state in the nation to have an inclusive community-based service system for people with developmental disabilities.

This manual is intended to assist the many audiences who participate in life planning, including case managers, vocational counselors, service providers, the people who are the focus of the planning, and their friends, families, neighbors, and co-workers. It includes various steps and procedures for building a personal vision of the future and outlines strategies and examples for getting there. I hope it will be helpful. Good luck!

Dale DiLeo
Training Resource Network
August, 1994

I

Service Plans: Beyond Programs

Many of us have discovered how people with disabilities contribute to our lives as friends, teachers, co-workers, and neighbors. We have seen how people's expectations have grown when they come to know an individual as a person first. They then experience directly what a person can accomplish, learn, and contribute.

But these changes have come slowly. Individuals with disabilities still generally are perceived as different by most people in our culture. These perceived differences tend to focus on negative images, and can be exaggerated by labels, intrusive programs, and the trappings of a human service system.

As a result, persons who have been labeled have found their lives restricted socially, economically, and culturally. Often, they have few opportunities to meet a variety of people who share their goals and interests.

Yet we all rely on our own communities and social network to achieve many of our life goals. It thus becomes critically important to open up avenues for persons to belong to their communities, meet others and develop lasting relationships, and achieve self-fulfillment and respect as people with something to contribute.

✦ Services Can Isolate People

People with severe disabilities have in particular arbitrarily been congregated and isolated from everyone else. A service system of special schools, institutions, or training programs that specialize in a disability has translated to limiting access to a diversity of relationships. This restricts the peer groups of these individuals to other persons subject to the same low expectations, with no other reason for being together than sharing a label, sometimes unfairly assigned.

Service plans in the past have been one contributor to the labeling process. In order to justify services, many plans initially focused on labels, deficiencies, and challenges. These were then translated to "treatment" strategies designed to remediate deficiencies.

The application of behavior technology enabled service staff to reduce life domains where change was desired into more achievable "learnable bits" of activities. Unfortunately, these also

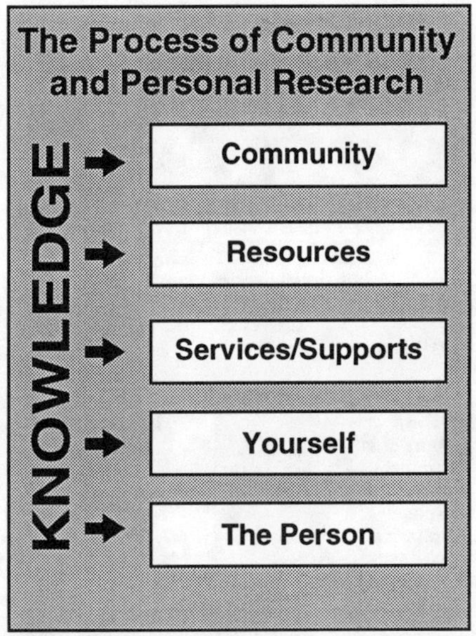

Before you can assist someone with a disability with services, you should be knowledgeable about a range of information. This includes your own resources and expectations, those of the individual to be served, and the attitudes, supports, and resources of the different communities with which the person will be involved.

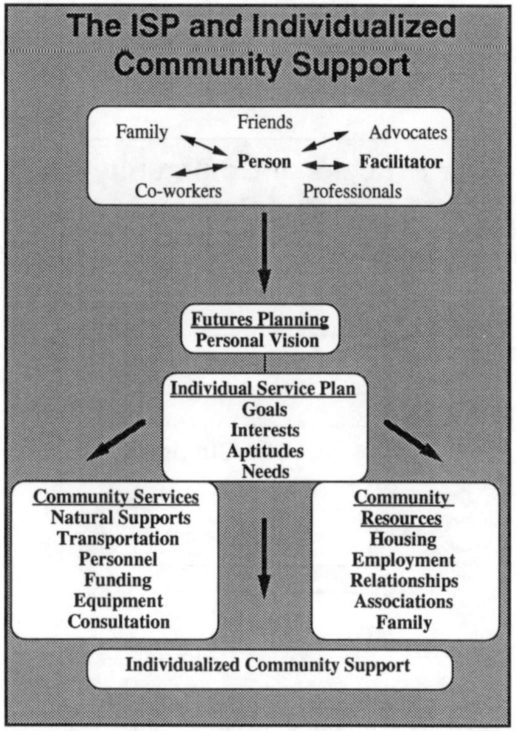

The ISP is developed based on a partnership with a service facilitator and the individual with a disability. They bring together a team of persons who can assist in developing and providing support for the individual to realize a desired quality of life. The outcome of this planning should be individualized community support.

tended to be simplistic and narrow objectives that became ends in themselves.

This approach meant that individuals with disabilities found themselves in very specialized programs that were organized around groups of people who shared perceived deficits. Lists of eligibility criteria and readiness skills were drawn up for people to master in order to move into a new level of specialized programming. Since they rarely moved, they unfortunately spent their lives in preparation for living a life in the community – a life few ever realized.

✦ Services That Support Community Inclusion

Another way to view services is to design them specifically around each person. Rather than "placing" people into existing rigid programs, we assist people with supports in ways that will improve their lives in directions each person dictates.

Supported employment is an example of an emerging service system for people with disabilities. It focuses on helping people to achieve a sense of social belonging through providing and supporting job opportunities in community settings designed around an individual. This is indeed different from traditional vocational services, which tend to try to make someone change to "get better."

Supported employment, like all community-based service, is really part of a *social movement*. It represents inclusion into the fabric of community, rather than segregating out a particular group of people for "specialized life treatment." A large part of that fabric is where we live, work, and recreate, and the people who are with us.

This philosophy of community inclusion is based on the concept of *normalization*, or *social role valorization* (Wolfensberger, 1972). In simple terms, it means "using supports, experiences, and environments that promote positive relationships, personal behaviors, and individual characteristics and roles that a community will value in a person" (DiLeo, 1993).

✦ Individual Needs Can Be Met through Natural Supports

When individuals with disabilities identify certain goals in their lives, assistance to help them reach such goals can take many forms. One way is to provide the kinds of services previously described. These approaches rely on formal assistance with home living, getting a job, communicating, or some other aspect of life.

But not all assistance need be formal. Informal supports from friends, co-workers, family, and other community members and organizations can also be helpful. These types of supports are called *natural supports*. Natural supports can be a particularly powerful way for people to realize the kind of lifestyle that more formal supports seem unable to provide.

✦ Individualized Supports Based on Accomplishments

To really be of assistance to individuals who have been denied life opportunities, we need to begin by learning about each person–his or her dreams, interests, skills, and aptitudes. Only after we discover some of the uniqueness of a person (truly knowing a person takes a lifetime and still brings surprises), can we try to plan supports and directions with and for him or her.

These supports should be drawn from natural community opportunities wherever possible, in ways that contribute to the person's personal growth and reputation. John O'Brien (1987) defined five essential service accomplishments for people with disabilities:

- sharing places
- making choices
- developing skills
- developing a positive reputation
- building relationships with others.

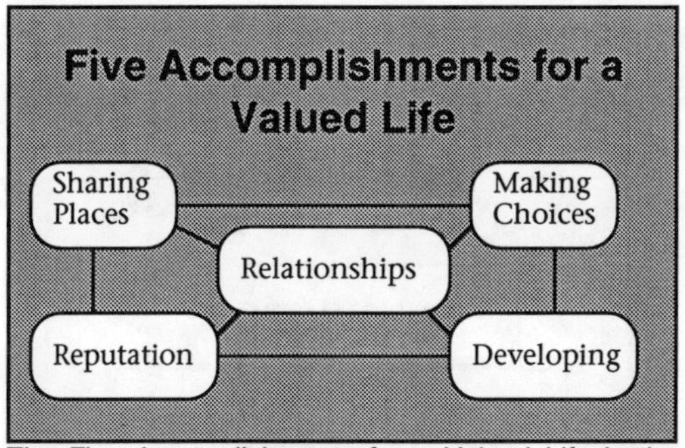

The Five Accomplishments for a Valued Life in the Community for Individuals with Disabilities (John O'Brien, 1986)

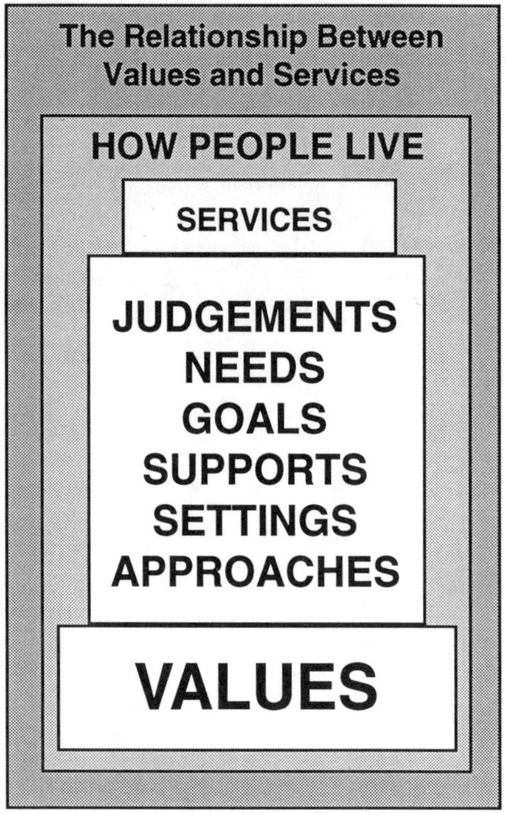

Values drive the judgements made about what people need, help shape opinions about future goals for the person, and determine how services get designed. Ultimately, attitudes impact how people with disabilities live, work, and recreate.

✦ The Individual Service Plan

Individual Service Plans (ISPs) have evolved to serve many functions for many different people and agencies. Because of this, there is often confusion about what an ISP is.

First and foremost, an ISP spells out the supports and strategies both needed and desired by an individual that would significantly improve his or her quality of life. The plan is developed based on what the person communicates, along with input from family, friends, and advocates, with the advice of service professionals. It is based on the person's life dreams, interests, capacities, and desires.

All states require that each person who receives state-funded services have such a plan detailing what those services and supports will be and what they will accomplish.

An ISP should:

- consist of comprehensive information from the person's life;
- be used as a flexible guide;
- place more importance on services that make sense in relation to a person's life than on predicting failure or success;
- not be reliant on norm-referenced tests to prove readiness; and
- involve and empower the individual, family and friends rather than relying solely on professional judgement (Callahan, 1991).

Notice that this plan derives from the individual and is not placed upon the person by service professionals. The way in which this plan is developed, what is included, and how it is monitored, will be addressed in this manual.

Like people, ISPs are constantly evolving. New ideas and planning techniques will continually change this process.

✦ Values That Shape ISPs

Our values and attitudes about planning services will influence and often determine what types of supports are offered to people and how they are delivered. This in turn helps shape the day-to-day life of someone with a disability. For this reason, it is important to clearly state preferred values. The following are eleven statements associated with the development and implementation of high quality ISPs:

Person-Centered Services

The person who receives services should be the central driving force in determining the kinds of supports, training, settings, and activities that are utilized.

Focus on Capacities

Individuals should be provided opportunities to develop and maintain skills of interest and use in their lives by discovering and expressing their unique gifts and capacities.

Individuality

People should be served as unique individuals with varying interests and aptitudes. They should not be grouped together on the basis of label, functioning level, or convenience of support.

Choice

Persons should receive options related to their interests and desires in life in order to exercise control and autonomy over the direction of their lives.

Respect

Services should be delivered in a dignified and age-appropriate way to enhance an individual's reputation.

Participation

People should have the opportunity to participate actively in all life pursuits of interest.

Social Connections

People should have access to diverse individuals in social contexts in order to build friendships, working relationships, and networks of individuals who share interests, settings, or other commonalities.

Community Settings with Minimal Intrusion

Services should be designed to support people in their pursuit of a quality life in natural settings and in ways that minimize artificiality or restrictiveness.

"Friends never feel they must fix you ..."
Bob Perske

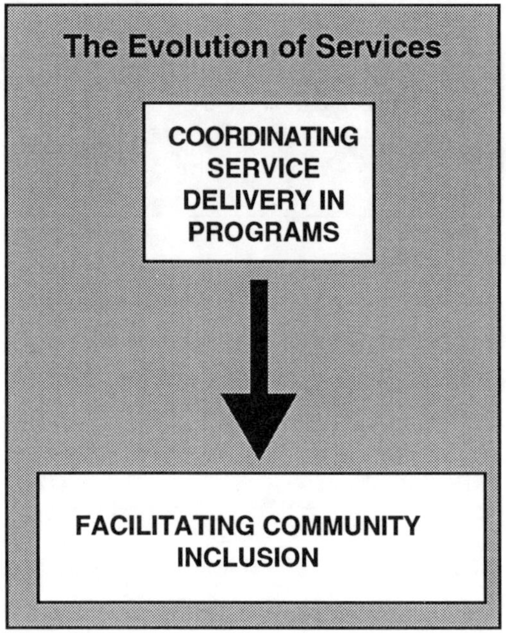

The traditional role of the individual who assists persons with disabilities to realize a better quality of life has evolved from placement into human service programs to a much broader scope of facilitating networks, relationships, and resources for community inclusion.

Holistic Life Support

Efforts to provide a holistic and integrated life support should be made. Individuals should have consistent service and community opportunities that connect to the fabric of work, home, social, and recreational needs.

Non-Intrusive, Effective Services

Existing natural supports should be used for training and ongoing support whenever possible. The use of artificial training or behavior programs should be minimized. Teaching techniques that may convey poor images, stigma, or devalued status should not be used. Specialized jargon from the disability field should be minimized.

At all times, the community culture should be respected and integrated into the support network for the individual to succeed. Use of accommodations, technology, or other environmental modifications should be explored.

Confidentiality

Individuals have a right to privacy and the confidential treatment of their lives, plans, services, and other matters.

✦ An Evolving Role for People Who Help Persons with Disabilities

The roles of people who assist persons with disabilities in their life planning are evolving. The values listed previously lead to activities that support a facilitation approach rather than a traditional care-giving one.

The following list illustrates this facilitation role. While the list may seem lengthy, it should not represent an overwhelming task. Rather, facilitators of a quality community life set individual priorities from within these strategies to accomplish the most important goals for each individual they support (Knoll and Ford, 1987).

Coming to Know the Individual and Helping to Plan Life Goals

- Meet informally with the individual to discuss life plans and review experiences, skills, and desires.
- Meet with key people who know the person well.
- Visit prior settings where the person spent time.

• Spend quality time together.
• Hire consultants when needed to evaluate specific areas such as behavior or physical therapy needs.
• Meet with the person to review reports.
• Respond to the directions provided by the person.
• Develop a "road map" to reach the realization of the life plan.

Developing Community Connections

• Meet with people in their homes to review their living situations or personal finances.
• Visit job sites when appropriate and be introduced to employers/co-workers; visit during break/lunch.
• Plan with the individual to attend community events.
• Go places together.
• Do community research–read local newspapers and visit local neighborhoods.
• Find community persons with whom to connect.
• Visit someone as a friend.
• Make community relations and educational visits.
• Make contacts with generic services to connect people in associations of interest, such as women's clubs and hobby groups.
• Help renew old acquaintances for people.
• Set up a church-based group for relationship building.
• Develop local transportation networks.
• Develop volunteer opportunities in community settings.

Advocacy

• Make calls/visits to state agencies for funding.
• Ask people to meet to help respond to crises needs.
• Provide assistance to individuals and their landlords or employers during difficult times.
• Be a positive role model in communities.
• Develop non-traditional service supports that are individualized.
• Help others to "let go" to reduce dependency.
• Provide/seek representation when needed through the legal system,

> **"Because it is so infrequently the case that excluded people and their families are able to overcome the barriers of service and incorporate themselves into community life, we have found that the most frequently successful incorporation has taken place as a result of people who have assumed a special responsibility to guide excluded people out of service into the realms of community life."**
>
> John McKnight

> "An effective facilitator knows how to build on the existing resources within communities and within people without waiting for something totally foreign to be injected that offers the often false promise of 'saving the day.' "
>
> Pat Beeman, George Ducharme, Beth Mount

guardianship, etc.

- Reduce overcommittment on outside personal decision-making and educate those responsible for trusts, guardianship, or representative-payees.
- Represent and support the individuals' view of their needs with funders, agencies, and outside services.

Quality Assurance

- Talk to providers of service.
- Make site visits with providers of service to observe and review documentation.
- Visit each person's home and support personnel to review life services.
- Make phone calls to providers of service to check agreements and follow-through.
- Ask each individual about satisfaction with services.
- Educate yourself about the range of options by networking with others.

Brokering Services

- Provide connections to unpaid, natural supports that exist in the community.
- Purchase time-limited specialty supports such as occupational or physical therapy.
- Develop a "community connection plan."
- Provide information on life plan goals for vendor service contracts.

Family Support

- Make phone calls to exchange information.
- Spend time with each family at home to review services.
- Meet with those who provide residential supports.
- Develop supports for siblings.
- Provide education by explaining options, giving examples, conveying visions, providing materials, and systems orientation.
- Link family to family and develop forums for networking.
- Link to professional advocates/educational advocates for families with younger children.
- Support each family through frustrating times.
- Provide informal counseling.

- When possible, help families to purchase their own services and supports.
- Offer assistance for families whose family member with a disability is at home.
- Help to re-unify/connect dispersed families.
- Assist families with estate planning.

Administrative

- Maintain logs and other needed documentation.
- Confer with funding/benefits technicians.
- Develop plans/timelines.
- Prioritize goals and activities.
- Disperse information – mail notes, minutes, correspondence.
- Collaborate with others for ideas, brainstorms, advice, and support.

✦ Summary

Being present in the community, either working on a job, shopping downtown, or living in a neighborhood, seems a large step forward for many individuals with disabilities. But physical integration alone, while necessary, is incomplete by itself. Social integration does not automatically follow. There are many people who are in "integrated" environments who are actively working and yet are very lonely.

Social equality is a matter of respect and participation in all aspects of a culture. It does not mean that a person gets treated like everyone else. It means that differences are considered, accommodated for, and channelled in the most productive and meaningful ways.

An important role of support staff is to utilize a service plan to assist people who need supports to achieve their preferred lifestyles in unique, personal ways. The plan should be a respectful document, based on personalized services that are integrated, meaningful, and aimed at enhancing each person's life.

Social equality occurs when a disability is not the prominent feature of a person. It recedes into the background as one among many facets, and it does not block inclusion into important aspects of the culture.

II

Assessment: Learning about a Person's Life Goals

Before any effort to develop a plan for services begins, it is absolutely necessary to first learn as much as possible about the individual to be served. One of the challenges in accomplishing this with individuals with a disabilities is that they often have had limited opportunities to explore their full potential. As a result, we often can only guess at the possibilities for their future.

Also, people who have had limited life experiences often are unaware of the range of choices before them. It is hard to discover interests when people have not had diverse interactions with environments, activities, and other people.

In addition, some individuals with disabilities have difficulty with communication. This requires effort and sensitivity to learn when a person is motivated, happy, involved, or disinterested. If language is not easily used, then these personal states may be communicated by expression, behavior, attentiveness, or other means.

✦ Traditional Testing Has Proven Limited

In the past, states and agencies mandated "professional testing" in order to gather information about the individual. This most often was done through formalized evaluation tools. Many times the results of this initial testing created a diagnostic label for an individual. A disability label often produces the unfortunate result of stereotypes and expectations for poor performance.

Testing also has practical limitations. Tests by themselves are generally inadequate to assess people's capabilities and life needs.

Testing takes a slice of performance at one fixed time in one setting. Usually the judgement of the examiner is needed to determine the response, particularly in evaluating people with significant difficulties in communication. Yet the examiner is seldom familiar with or close to the person being tested. This may mean that much of a person's life may be determined from an inadequate testing experience.

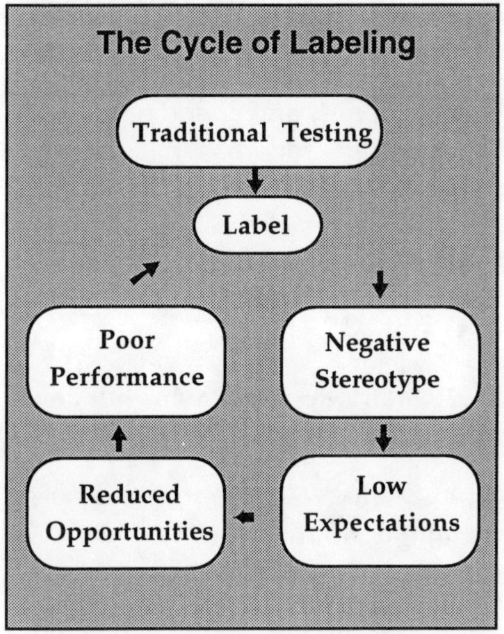

A self-fulfilling prophecy of few opportunities can occur when traditional testing institutes a label for an individual with a disability.

Sources of Information for Assessment

1. Interview and spend time with the person to receive services. Visit their home, job, day program, and social places. Invest time informally, not as a "sample observation," but rather as a human experience.

2. Interview and visit with the person's family.

3. Speak with friends and colleagues whom the individual or family has identified.

4. Meet with professionals who have worked with the person.

5. Hire professionals to assess specific life areas such as health, nutrition, employment, communication, and movement.

6. Research past records for information, other contacts, and previous history.

The concept of test-defined competency implies a permanent ceiling of capability, rather than individual lifelong development. No label, behavior, test result, or diagnosis can clearly define potential and predict functioning.

Instead, these classifications tend to be more predictive of service environments and relationships in which people will be placed. These are based on assumed needs and generally low expectations. Tragically, these settings are often far less challenging, normalized, and prestigious. This in turn restricts development, potential, and status.

Formalized tests can provide a glimpse of information about the individual under certain conditions, particularly when specific questions are asked and expertise is sought. These data may be useful and even important. But they should never be viewed in isolation and out of the context of the person's whole life.

✦ Moving from Deficiency to Competency

Too many assessments consist solely of checklists of skills we expect people to have. These expectations come from such things as age and development, social standards of behavior, or analysis of component skills related to areas of life such as work or home living.

After testing people, we compare their performance to our lists. We then highlight the differences found, listing them as "needs" or "deficiencies."

If there is a pattern to the lists, we apply a label or diagnosis to the performance. This label may actually have practical uses for research or planning about *groups* of people who happen to share certain kinds of needs. By providing a common language, labels allow us to understand what we mean when we talk about a certain group.

The downside is that a label can work against an *individual* in powerful ways. Language can stereotype a person by reducing expectations of his or her performance or potential due to preconceived notions of what labels such as "profoundly retarded" or "behaviorally disordered" mean.

✦ Gathering Information about the Person

There are several strategies that may be applied to conduct a meaningful personal life assessment. These are:

- Research previously recorded information, but guard against the potential for flawed or outdated material.
- Spend time together in a variety of environments.
- Review materials, books, videos, or other media to learn about interests.
- Talk with the person (see list at right).
- Speak with those involved with the individual whom the person has either indicated or granted permission to see.
- Seek professional evaluations for specific life domains.
- Accompany the individual on community outings.

20 Questions to Ask to Begin a Personal Life Assessment

There is a large variety of questions to pursue. Here are 20 to get you started.

1. What is (your) (the person's) dream in life?

2. What is (your) (the person's) favorite kind of work?

3. Where do (you) (the person) want to live?

4. When are (you) (the person) most happy?

5. Where/when are (you) (the person) motivated?

6. What are some places (you) (the person) would like to be in?

7. How do (you) (the person) know how to ask for help, tell others about your needs, or problem solve?

8. What experiences have (you) (the person) had in the past that influence you today?

9. What are (your) (the person's) work experiences?

10. What is going on in (your) (the person's) life outside of work?

11. Are (you) (the person) feeling well?

12. What are some things (you) (the person) would like to do?

13. Who are some people (you) (the person) would like to meet, see, or do things with?

14. What are some of the things (you) (the person) do best?

15. What makes (you) (the person) unique?

16. Who are the people (you) (the person) are connected to?

17. How do (you) (the person) learn best?

18. What kinds of accomplishments are most important to (you) (the person)?

19. What special considerations are needed for (you) (the person) to be at your best?

20. What other questions should I be asking?

These questions should only be a starting point in the exploration of the life and personality of an individual. If the person is unable to comprehend them, rephrase the questions in ways that the person can understand.

> **"This set of accomplishments (community presence, choice, participation, respect, and competence) frames the basic question of personal futures planning: 'How can we identify constructive actions which will improve the quality of life experiences for the person we are concerned about?' "**
>
> John O'Brien

This early investment of time is important to know and understand the individual. It pays off a hundredfold when you are planning, coordinating, and monitoring services for the person.

✦ Person-Centered Planning

An alternative to assessing needs through testing and labeling is to help facilitate a person-centered approach to planning. This process has been described in many ways, including:

- *Personal Futures Planning* (O'Brien, 1987)
- *MAPS* (Forest and Snow, 1987; Vandercook and York, 1988)
- *Circles of Support* (Mount, 1987)
- *Essential Lifestyle Planning* (O'Brien and Lovett, 1993).

All these planning strategies share the belief that the best way to discover a person's interests, needs, experiences, and aptitudes is through a sensitive exploration of life history, experiences, and social relationships. There is a focus on ability rather than on deficits.

Planning meetings should be a balance of professionals and non-professionals, but primarily include people who care about and are committed to the individual. A loosely conducted but structured and well-facilitated meeting process is recommended. Record on a flip chart accomplishments, relationships, resources, and potential ideas relating to career, home, and other domains.

✦ Personal Futures Planning

John O'Brien (1987) described an orderly process for working toward a desirable future for an individual with a disability called personal futures planning. A team works with the person to decide on a schedule of activities and supports that will organize available resources to move toward that future.

The process generates information by determining:

- the quality of the person's present life experiences
- what is changing for the person or

in the surrounding environment that is likely to influence the quality of the person's life
- the most important threats and opportunities to better quality life experiences for the person
- the image of a desirable future for the person
- the most critical barriers to moving toward the desirable future described
- how to effectively manage these critical barriers and move toward the defined future
- the next steps
- the necessary changes in the capabilities of the service system

✦ McGill Action Planning System (MAPS)

The McGill Action Planning System (MAPS) (Forest and Snow, 1987; Vandercook and York, 1988) is an affirming process that assists a team to creatively dream and plan. Its aim is to produce results that will further the inclusion of individuals with labels into the activities, routines, and environments of their peers in their communities. Although designed with students and school environments in mind, the process is functional with any age or setting.

The MAPS planning typically occurs in one or two sessions. Participants are arranged in a half circle, with the facilitator positioned at the open end of the circle. The information and ideas generated come from the following seven questions, and are recorded on large chart paper:

- *What is the individual's history?*
This comes from a discussion of milestones and significant events.
- *What is the dream for the individual?*
The team envisions beyond the current reality.
- *What is your nightmare?*
This anticipates situations that the team must work to keep from happening.
- *Who is the person?*
The participants are asked to think of words that describe the individual. There are no right or wrong words. Participants take turns going around the circle until all thoughts have been expressed.

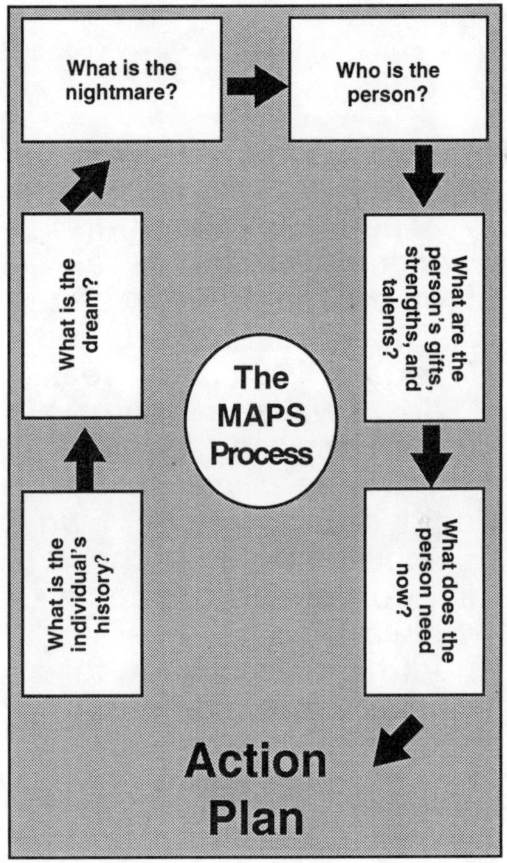

"The circle of support concept was first developed by Judith Snow and Marsha Forest in Toronto, Canada in 1980 ... to break down walls that kept Judith imprisoned in the institution ... eventually Judith moved into her own apartment ...With the support of caring people who were a part of her life, Judith made a vision for her life into a reality."

Beth Mount,
Pat Beeman,
George Ducharme

• *What are the individual's strengths, gifts, and abilities?*

This requires identifying and building upon the individual's capacities.

• *What are the individual's needs?*

This provides an opportunity for team members to identify needs from each of their unique perspectives.

• *What would the individual's ideal day look like and what must be done to make it happen?*

The MAPS process provides a common vision for team members that enables them to be supportive and effective in furthering the integration of individuals with disabilities.

✦ Circles of Support

A circle of support is a group of people who meet regularly to help a person with a disability accomplish personal goals (Mount, Beeman, Ducharme, 1988). If the individual is unable to reach these goals working alone, he or she asks a number of people to work with her or him to overcome obstacles and to open doors to new opportunities. The circle members provide support to the person and take action on her or his behalf.

The members of a circle of support usually include friends, family members, co-workers, neighbors, and sometimes service providers. The majority of people are not paid to be there – they are involved because they care about the focus person and have made a commitment to work together on his or her behalf. Circles in no way exclude paid service providers, but the majority of members are non-paid, typical community people.

The person and his or her spokesperson determine every aspect of the circle including membership, setting, image of the future, and frequency of meetings. The circle does not "belong to the system," but depends on the local community for its effectiveness.

The circle process follows the guidelines for personal futures planning as outlined before:

- discover capacities
- find directions for change
- generate strategies
- make commitments
- reflect on what is being learned together

✦ Essential Lifestyle Planning

Essential lifestyle planning (O'Brien and Lovett, 1993) was developed to assist people in moving from institutions into the community. This process revolves around discovering three sets of core values from the person and those who know him or her well (see box at right).

These values are listed under the following categories:

- Non-negotiables
- Strong preferences
- Highly desirables

Like personal futures planning, these discoveries help shape a desired future life for the individual. This information is then used to develop an agreement between those representing the person and the community service providers who will help the person.

Supports and services can then better account for the person's disability, while at the same time helping him or her achieve a desired lifestyle. This is because the plan is based on a core vision as well as a set of preferences (with different priorities) for the future. Typically, an independent person directs the process.

✦ Utilize Information from Different Life Domains

There are so many aspects to a person's life that it is easy to miss a significant area that may play a part in the planning process. Therefore, it is important to explore all the domains within life to arrive at a more complete understanding of the person. Some of these might include:

- leisure
- significant life events
- expectations for the future
- social life
- school and education
- family life
- home life
- neighborhood community
- skills and capacities
- communication
- health
- unique support needs
- learning style
- mobility/transportation

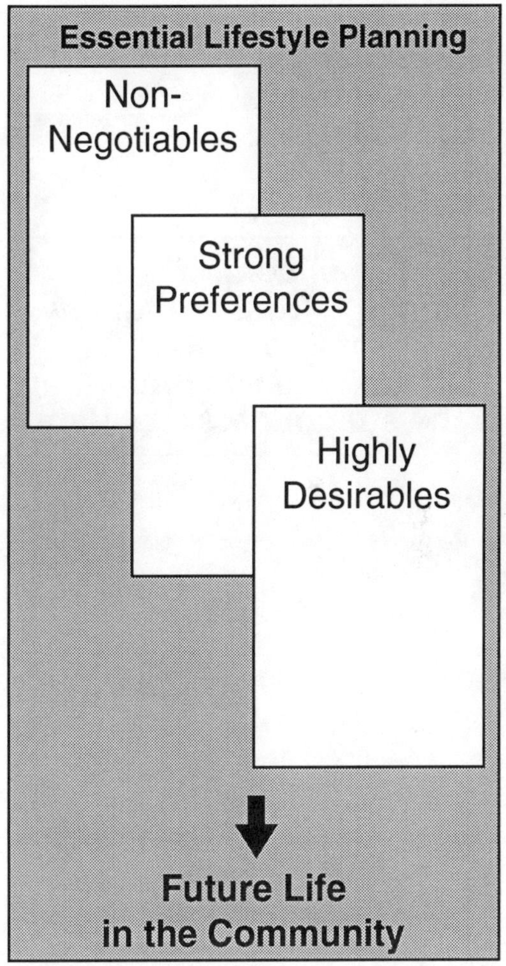

A real person must emerge from the totality of information. An individual is more than the sum of personal data.

✦ Synthesize Information into a Coherent Picture

Gathering large amounts of information about a person will be of little use until the findings are placed in a context that is unified. A person must emerge from all the bits of knowledge learned. Since a person is more than the sum of data, care must be taken to holistically convey impressions of the uniqueness of a total individual. To do this, it will be helpful to:

- describe what you and others have found
- synthesize information
- make some guesses about what the person wants, likes, needs, and what he or she is trying to communicate through his or her behavior
- ask, "What else should I know?"
- stay involved; personal information will change and evolve
- make an outline/notes that you will use to write a personal profile

✦ Summary

There are many traditional tools to assess individuals for the purpose of finding their deficiencies and applying a label. These tools are not as effective in helping people to plan personal futures based on their interests, skills, and dreams. A better process is to discover information about the person as an individual and build a fuller understanding of his or her life goals.

III

Developing Personal Profiles

Good service planning begins by exploring and discovering over time each person's interests, skills, gifts, and experiences as described earlier. This information is used to build a personal profile. What we learned about an individual through "assessment" is synthesized into an understandable life story – a document that succinctly describes the person and his or her life.

The information should be enough to give readers unfamiliar with the individual a sense of where to begin their education. A written profile need not be long – it might only be about one or two typed pages.

Sample Profile Excerpts: Robert

... Robert is a pleasant, likeable 22-year-old gentleman with a positive disposition and a willingness to help others. He is very sociable and polite, and likes to please people. He lives with his family and is currently seeking a job. He attends a vocational program and is on a waiting list for residential services.

... Robert has Down Syndrome. Like all people, each person with Down Syndrome has unique capabilities. Drawing and writing are two of Robert's talents. He also enjoys card games, watching movies, and working on clerical tasks. He does not like idle time.

... Robert learns best when he has verbal directions and a model. He is motivated by work itself and receiving praise from those he cares about. Close people in his life include his parents, brothers, and George, a staff person in his day program.

... Robert enjoys trying new things and is very capable of learning new jobs and skills. Once he is familiar with a job, he tends to change his performance to his own "style." Usually, his finished work is still the same, but despite his ingenuity, his new procedure is often not efficient and increases his margin of error. When this becomes a problem, it requires a difficult process of relearning the original method.

✦ Portrayal and Language

The language that has generally been used to describe individuals with disabilities has been the language of difference, stigma, and deficiency. Many professionals have been trained to assess deficiencies (see Chapter II), and to use words and labels to describe an individual.

These labels, such as "severely/profoundly retarded," "low function-

Sample Profile Excerpts: Robert

... Robert's persistence in modifying methods of work borders on stubbornness at times, according to those who work with him. Yet his accomplishments are impressive. He is neat, precise, and orderly. He constantly cleans and reorganizes his work area. According to his parents, he can "fold clothes and make his bed to the accuracy of a ruler!" They describe him as very independent and a fast worker. At home, it is his responsibility to keep his room neat and clean, and he takes pride in this.

... While Robert seems to enjoy his day program, it mostly consists of sub-contract assembly and clerical work, some of which is practice material. Robert and those who know him best have asked for assistance in obtaining a real job for him. The staff who work with him report that he enjoys working so much that he is usually not interested in break times. They also feel he requires close supervision and needs constant support to not change task procedures. He has not had many opportunities for experiencing real employment, despite his motivation for work.

ing," or "non-compliant" have negative connotations. They are so laden with stereotypes and misinformation that freely using them might:

- cause a subtle negative reaction (conscious or subconscious) by the reader
- set up low expectations of performance
- cause an individual to be perceived in inaccurate ways

✦ Use Everyday, Respectful Language

When writing a personal profile based on the information gathered earlier, begin by describing the person as a unique individual with personality, skills, and interests to understand. Try describing the person to someone who has never met him or her and would enjoy the experience. Use everyday words about personality traits, appearance, and other qualities that make this person who he or she is.

Minimize the use of human service jargon. For instance, instead of saying someone is "non-compliant," describe how the individual might express frustration or prefer not to take direction. Instead of saying he or she has "inappropriate social behaviors," describe what sort of social experiences the individual needs to experience in order to improve his or her social graces. Rather than saying someone is "low-functioning," describe what the person is capable of doing with and without various supports.

Follow the guidelines for language usage as set out by advocacy groups such as The Association for Persons with Severe Handicaps. Use descriptors of disability that follow "person first" (person with mental retardation rather than mentally retarded person). Do not refer to a group of people as a disability (the retarded). Do not use dated terms such as "educable" or "trainable."

Sample Profile Excerpts: Sharon

... Sharon is an outgoing 36-year-old woman who recently moved to a duplex in town. She shares her home with two male roommates. Four individuals who have developmental disabilities live in the other side of the building.

... Sharon has adjusted well to her new home. She lives in a renovated "suite" in the basement. Her living area includes a bedroom and an additional room. She takes a great deal of pride in her rooms and chooses to spend much of her time organizing her things. She has two closets, which enables her to keep her many possessions fairly organized. Since she moved, her living space is much more neat and less cluttered.

... Sharon's favorite chore at home is cooking, although she is active in many varied tasks. In her spare time, she enjoys shopping, swimming, singing, and dancing. She likes having her hair and make-up done and going to church. Other interests include movies, parties, picnics, card games, camping, and playing basketball.

... Sharon is currently employed part-time at Smith & Company, working on a variety of clerical tasks. This is her second position within six months. While she did well at her previous job, she occasionally demanded immediate attention and was loud in doing so. She lost her job when she entered a restricted area. She also currently does landscaping and housekeeping to supplement her income. She does her best work when she is in community settings with good role models who enjoy her company.

Sample Profile Excerpts: Sharon

... Since Sharon has had difficulty with communication, she is participating in therapy to help her make more eye contact, use sign and line drawings to convey her message, and to be more accepting of constructive criticism.

... The people in her life are pleased she has more control of her tendency to tear bits of her clothing. This has decreased to less than one occasion per month. She continues to need assistance in order to use the bathroom during the night, and also likes to visit the refrigerator for a snack several times during the evening.

... Social relationships are very important to Sharon, and she takes them very seriously. With some assistance, she has started to write home to her mother weekly. She is strongly attached to Bonnie, a support person at her home, and to Roberta, who helps her with her job. Sharon is an extremely affectionate and outgoing person who has shown the ability to be socially responsible when given the right opportunities.

✦ Describe Disability Functionally

Being open and honest about an individual and his or her needs for support and accommodation is critical. Many times ISPs serve to support eligibility for certain services. Also, good communication is the basis for developing successful supports for an enhanced quality of life.

• Begin by talking about capabilities and interests:

"Mr. King is a very reliable and hard worker who is very accurate in his production, and ..."

"Ms. Casey is a very sociable person who enjoys music, sports ..."

• Cite specific life experiences:

"He worked in an office before at C.J. Jones, where he was responsible for filing, copying, and other clerical work ..."

• Introduce an individual's needs in the context of performance. An individual's disability is best described in terms of additional supports or modifications needed to function successfully. Rather than use a label, describe those supports:

"For her to do well on the job, she needs ..."

"In order to move around in the community, he uses a wheelchair to ..."

"It takes her a bit longer to learn a routine at first, but once ..."

If there is a reason to use a specific label (for funding eligibility, or because the label relates to the functional description) state the label but add qualifying descriptors that make this person unique:

"She has cerebral palsy, which means something very different for each person. For instance, she is able to ..."

Hiding previous or potential concerns or overestimating performance can also set up an individual for failure. The key is to talk about what is needed for success for the individual in specific terms.

Sample Profile Excerpts: Lloyd

... Lloyd is very aware of his environment. He responds to changes in sounds, people, facial expressions, body language, and to his own name. He is able to follow three-step verbal directions.

... Lloyd responds best to verbal interactions when you get his attention first. He also understands many routines and familiar words, such as mealtime and work. He responds to "yes/no" and "do you want" questions through facial expressions, (smiles) body language (moves around in his wheelchair), and by vocalizing "yes" and shaking his head "no" or ignoring you.

...He will respond to simple "what" questions by answering yes/no, reaching/pointing, or taking you to what he wants. People familiar with Lloyd can understand him most of the time. Lloyd likes to be in the middle of things, either helping out or partaking in activities. If people cannot understand what he is trying to communicate, he will either repeat the message or quit trying.

... Lloyd's primary means of transportation is his wheelchair as a result of the amputation of his right leg. He is able to propel his wheelchair using both hands within any wheelchair accessible environment. He also independently transfers to and from his chair, needing assistance to lock his brakes.

✦ What to Include

The following areas can be used as a guide and checklist for writing a personal profile. While there is no rigid formula, it is a good idea to think about each area to be certain you have fully explored the individual's life:

- Personality traits, age, defining physical features, and characteristics
- Places, activities, friends, pursuits, hobbies the person enjoys
- Social relationships with colleagues, friends, family, co-workers
- Personal history, including accomplishments and challenges faced
- Past and current living situations, with supports and arrangements needed and preferred, neighborhood and community
- Past and current employment, with supports and accommodations needed and preferred, job title, employer, skills used
- Significant life events, achievements, personal/social growth, new experiences and roles
- Learning style, competencies, skills
- Manner of communicating needs and choices
- Health, stamina, mobility, medical needs

✦ Summary

Any one person has a host of characteristics, experiences, and potential. Exploring these things first is more useful than boxing someone in with a label and the limitations it implies. This requires a discussion of specific individual support needs and an avoidance of letting the disability define the individual. It is important to use respectful language that honestly paints a complete picture of the person.

IV

Determining a Personal Future

We all have ideas about what we want to achieve in life and how we eventually want our lives to look. Sometimes these are vague visions of careers and lifestyles, other times they are more specific. Many times our life's goals relate to what we would like to change in our current situation. Today's relationships, living situations, careers, and other factors influence how we want the future to be.

People with disabilities are no different. Listening and learning about a person with a disability and discovering aspects about his or her personality are necessary first steps to helping the person to think about the future. Techniques for accomplishing this are described in Chapter II, Assessment: Learning about a Person's Life Goals.

How this information is unified into a personal profile was the topic of the previous section. A profile organizes information into a "snapshot" of an individual and most of what is important to him or her in life.

But without a coherent vision of where someone is heading, or a "personal future," it is hard to coordinate whatever supports might be needed along the way. Information gleaned from learning about a person should be thought about in context with prospective community settings, social situations, employment, recreation, and other pursuits. In this way, you can assist the individual to evolve a vision of the future with meaningful quality life opportunities of personal importance.

The sample document at right is a summary of a team's preliminary planning efforts around designing a career for an individual whose life dream included being meaningfully employed.

✦ Discover and Respect the Person's Aspirations and Life Dreams

All too often, an individual with a disability, or perhaps a parent or friend, has a vision that professionals or others dismiss as "unrealistic." How can he or she possibly be a singer, a boss, an artist, a doctor?

But immediate rejection of dreams, however seemingly unrealistic, denies people a means of communicating

Sample Futures Planning Worksheets

Favorite Places to Be:	***Personality***
McDonald's Visiting friends Shopping K-Mart Fun Spot Dunkin Donuts Adult Basic Educ. Church Camp Friendship YMCA	Outgoing Stubborn Humorous Sociable/friendly Positive attitude Affectionate Problem solver Seldom seeks help

Favorite Things to Do:	***Uniqueness***
Dining Camping out Visiting friends "Paperwork" Magazine/pictures Basketball/golf Strumming guitar Watch wrestling Play-acting Dancing Watching movies Being with people Boating	Dislikes being corrected Needs help with communicating Possessions are important: - Likes "office supplies" - Nice clothes - Cassettes

continued on next page

continued from previous page

Resources
Guardian receives SSI of $80/mo.
Friends: Fern, Jennifer, & Judy
Informal relationships

Communication
Picture-cards in wallet
Self created gestures
Acting

Work Experiences
Health club janitorial
Housecleaning
Webster Valve deburring
Road Crew - outside cleaning
ES Workshop assembly and packaging; loading/unloading

Career Brainstorms
Physical; not high paced
Recycling company
Salesman
Basketball coach
Inventory
Stocking
Material handling
Mover
Attendant - unloading cars
Hospital orderly
Schools - cafeteria, phys. ed. recess/bus monitor, paper, janitorial, library, office equipment manager
Health clubs - athletic instructor, equipment manager
Restaurants - waiter, dishwasher, busperson
Fast food positions
Yard work

Career Brainstorms II
Movie houses/TV projection assistant
Camps/resorts - activity coordinator
Acting Co./theater
Laundry/dry cleaning
Retail - clothes, office supply
State parks
Supermarkets - stock, material handling, bagging
Arcades - attendant
Farm work
Video store - inventory/returns
Library/book store- cataloging, logging periodicals, cleaning, check out, book binding

Accommodations
Communication
Structured tasks (check lists, co-worker support)
Flexibility

Potential Sites
Library
Post office/UPS
Dunkin Donuts
McDonalds
Jackson Star
Colonial Theater

Transportation
Service provider
Neighbors
If local, walk
Co-workers

Job Description
Work that relates to his interests: people, office-related, physical labor, acting/drama, helping people, greeting people

important information that should be respected. These dreams provide critical information on people's future paths and how this relates to their quality of life.

When considering life goals, think of how best to help the person *approach* the realization of a life's dream. For example, if an individual expresses a desire to be a musician, seek creative ways to vocationally enter a field in which music is involved. Working in a music store, in a theater, or at a radio station may help the individual be close to his or her dream.

Interest in a particular profession, even if the profession itself seems unrealistic, provides a pathway to connecting with the settings and trappings of a career.

✦ Use Future Planning Processes

The personal futures planning process described previously can be very helpful in developing an understanding about who the person is and what he or she needs. The approach guides people through essential activities that help describe a desirable future with the person. It also focuses on developing supports and responsibilities that will organize available resources to move toward that future.

Personal futures planning is not a magical process that provides quick answers. Sometimes it can be complicated and difficult. What people need can be very different from what they are presumed to need because of their disabilities.

The box at right contains an example of a futures statement for an individual with a disability.

Sample Futures Statement

Susan states that her dreams in life include being "on my own" and "my own boss," along with aspiring to be a professional singer. She would also like to have a boyfriend.

In the next few years, she will approach her dream of independence by moving from her group home and living in her own apartment in her home town. She will live either with a roommate of her choice who can help her with the apartment living skills she needs to learn, or with a paid attendant or staff.

She will pursue a career related to music, working up to full-time at prevailing wages in a setting with many other people who share her love of music. Her job will provide some of the autonomy she desires and should be near where she lives.

She will focus her personal growth in independent home living skills, particularly cooking. She will come to better appreciate the importance of good decisions in shopping, cooking, and eating in their relationship to health. She will also exercise to maintain a healthy weight.

Susan will also pursue her interests in movies, hiking, and music by expanding her social connections through community theater, friends at work and church, and joining a community nature club. Susan's family connections will be supported through letters, visits, and celebrations. Her relationships with her current friends will be supported and expanded, and she will hopefully meet a boyfriend whose companionship she enjoys.

✦ Considerations for Developing Futures Statements

A futures statement projects the "best guess" of where, what, and how the person, with the input of the people who care about him or her, wants to move forward in life. It should be a few well-written, brief paragraphs (about a half to full page at most). The statement should take into consideration the information gathered and summarized in the life domains of the personal assessment.

By writing a few succinct statements summarizing the person's vision in a number of life domains, the planning team provides a written context for choosing the strategies to realize that vision.

Some of these domains are the following:

✦ *Preferred Life Dreams*

What are the hopes, aspirations, and even life fantasies of the person and those involved who care about him or her?

✦ *Relationships/Belonging*

Who are the key people who will be involved and what will define their relationship?

✦ *Work*

What type of career, hours, position, location, setting, does the person prefer?

✦ *Living Arrangements*

Where will the person live? What type of home in what kind of setting? Describe roommates, family, neighborhood considerations, type of community (urban, suburban, rural, small town, etc.).

✦ *Personal Interests/ Leisure Pursuits*

How will the individual incorporate motivating interests and/or hobbies into meaningful activities and participation?

✦ *Personal Growth*

What kinds of competencies does the person wish and need to learn to realize the goals and future statements described?

✦ *Health*

What areas of healthy living will need support?

✦ *Special Considerations*

What are the unique aspects of this person that should be considered in projecting future life?

✦ Summary

A personal future is an evolving concept, so a service plan needs to be flexible as well. If the individual who is facilitating planning takes the time to invest up front in learning about the individual and her or his potential community, then long-term quality of life is much more likely.

V

Writing Service Plans Using Measurable Objectives

Once a person's team has listened, learned, and documented what it knows about an individual, the next step is to help the person project some concrete directions in his or her personal life. This starts with the personal futures statement discussed in the previous section.

Once thoughts are written down about future areas the person wants to change, develop, or maintain, the team may wish to build a "road map." This map will be the plan on how to get to the described vision.

A road map is a useful analogy. One can take many different routes to get to a goal. Some routes take longer, but may be more enjoyable along the way. Others are more direct and perhaps speedier.

The choice of routes is as important as the goal itself. Sometimes the journey matters even more than the realization of the goal. That is why we should take seriously the responsibility of developing specific service support objectives.

Performance and service objectives are part of a menu of individualized supports for a person. Public funders generally require written objectives as part of a person's plan.

✦ When to Use Objectives

Using measurable objectives as a road map can be helpful when the team wishes its members to be very specific about their responsibilities and to be accountable for their commitments. The elements of an objective are described at right.

Objectives work best when the person wishes to master precise actions, skills, or competencies. They are weakest around defining general quality of life statements, such as meaningful participation in community activities or social relationships.

This is because it is difficult to define social integration, meaningfulness, or quality of experiences satisfactorily. How do we objectively quantify a meaningful relationship? Can we truly measure the experience of an integrated community outing?

Although we can approximate these types of activities with various reports of data, it is challenging to realistically write a specific objective that is useful in this area.

There are instances when you can

When Objectives Are Effective Tools

Define objectives for services when the individual and the team desire:

- **accountability for services**
- **data on learning and performance**
- **documentation for funding**
- **precision to decide priorities and strategies**

What Makes Up an Objective?

There are many different ways of defining goals and objectives. Goals are usually thought of as general statements of what is expected in a particular life domain.

Objectives are more measurable, precise statements of expected achievement. Measurable objectives should include:

Subject
Person expected to act.

Action
An observable action verb that can be verified.

Conditions
What should be, might be, or needs to be present for the person to act.

Criteria
How the action will be measured and considered mastered.

approach this creatively. For example, an individual (or family member or staff person) involved may be able to "rate" his or her satisfaction with social life or community experiences by assigning a number from one to five. The composite score will approximately reflect the "quality" of those experiences over a given month, for instance. This might be helpful feedback, but realistically may not be a terribly valid or reliable measure of quality of life.

But when there are complex behavioral, vocational, or skill challenges, the use of *task analysis,* or reducing complicated sets of actions to more manageable bits of learning, can be helpful. Performance objectives allow support people to keep careful records on progress and growth. This can be helpful when there are many teachers, trainers, or other support people who move in and out of the person's life.

Another consideration is that sometimes perspective can be lost over time and across the many people who are involved with an individual who needs services. Objective data can provide important feedback, point to next steps, or indicate a need for a change in support strategy. Finally, when there are funding sources that require very careful documentation of service, performance objectives can be useful in tracking a record of service and progress.

✦ Context

Making good judgements about what a person will learn is difficult. Objectives are meaningless without some context to place them in. This is even more true if the objectives are small slices of a more complex behavior. Many times, the people providing service are new or unaware of the planning that preceded the development of an objective. All they may see is the objective itself.

To remind those who assist the individual, it is a good idea to state the overall meaning of the objective in a preamble statement, as in the sample performance objective on the previous page. This phrase will link the "slice" of behavior to the more meaningful life goal. A summary of how objectives should relate back to a person's life dream appears at right.

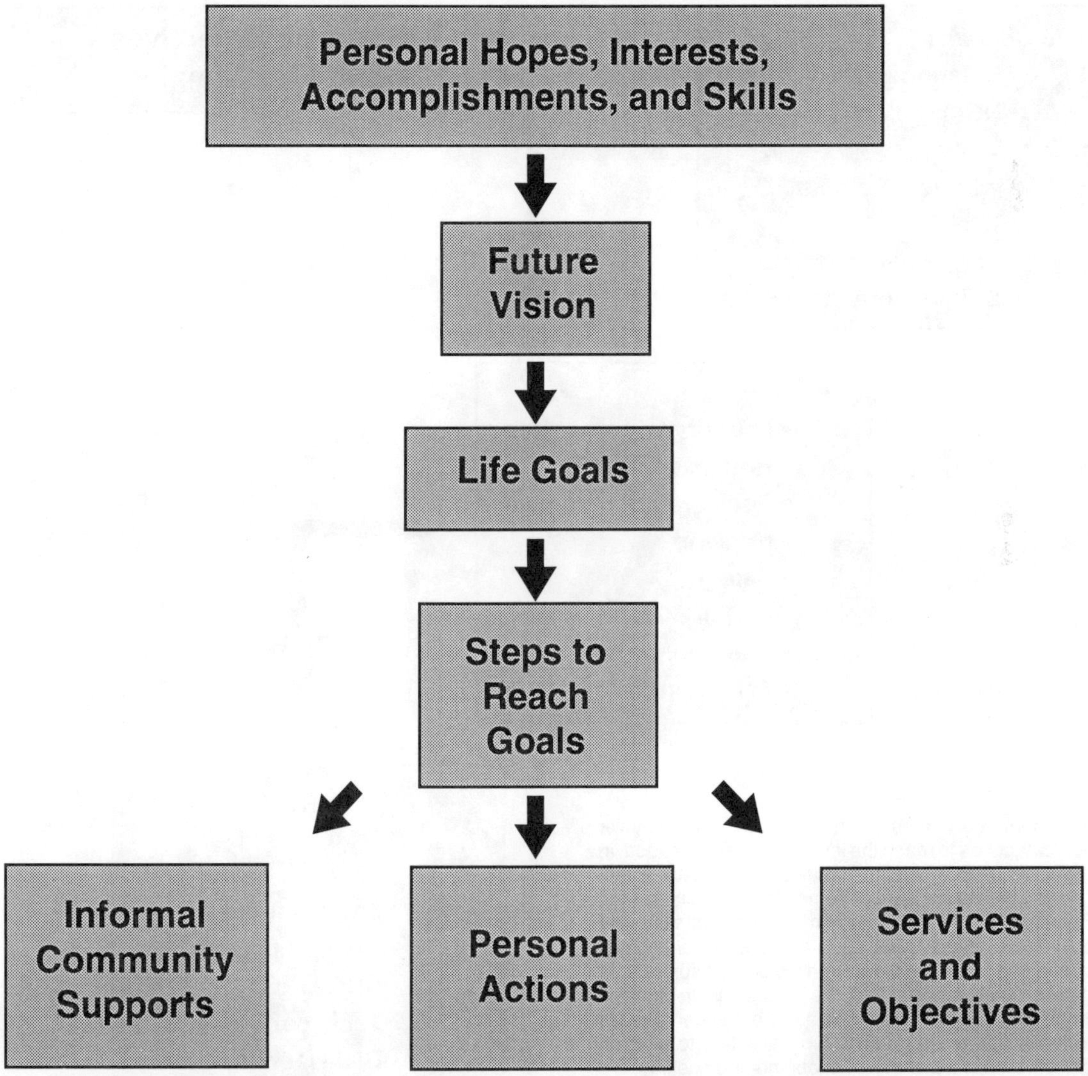

Selecting Objectives from Life Domains

BOX 1

Life Domains

- Relationships
- HOME LIVING →
- Work
- Interests/Leisure
- Health
- Personal growth
- Unique considerations

BOX 2

Home Living

- Laundry
- Housekeeping
- Social relationships
- Hygiene
- Safety
- NUTRITION →
- Transportation
- Telephone, etc.

BOX 3

Nutrition

- Meal planning
- SHOPPING →
- Food storage
- Meal preparation
- COOKING →
- Table setting
- Dishwashing, etc.

Each domain of interest can be further sliced into smaller sub-categories to reach the level of precision needed. In the example above, Life Domains (BOX 1) are listed, one of which is the area of home life. The Home Living Domain (BOX 2) can include many kinds of skills and activities to accomplish such as those listed above, depending on the individual and his or her future vision. If the planning team were to then focus on one of these, Nutrition (BOX 3), there still remains a number of areas to analyze before deciding which skill or task to focus an objective on. Two of these, shopping and cooking, are further analyzed on the next page.

✦ How to Choose Slices of Life Domains as Priorities

In many ways, setting life priorities is a presumptuous task for anyone other than the person himself or herself. For instance, knowing what to focus energy on when a person wishes to live in his or her own apartment depends a great deal on what the person already knows, what supports are in place, and what resources might be needed to get to the goal.

A combination of skill requirements, what the person can do, and his or her hopes, desires, and interests can lead to making good choices for objectives.

One exercise to help plan how to make these kind of decisions is to follow a *taxonomy*, or list of elements that together make up the competencies of a goal such as "living on your own." Each element of a goal can usually be broken down further into sub-areas, which in turn can be analyzed further into more components.

The level of precision and analysis needed for learning and accomplishment can then be chosen, taking into consideration what areas can be modified, supported, or done without. The most important concern will be the person's wishes and how they fit with his or her life goals. Other things to think about are likelihood of success, speed of learning, generalizability, and the functional nature of the skill.

A learning objective should be:

- achievable within a three-to-twelve month time frame
- a critical priority within the futures plan
- based on the person's interests and capacities

Another important consideration is to make the objective as global as possible within a domain while still enabling a person to accomplish it. Generally, the more specialized the objective, the less direct the life relevance.

An objective on "identifying coins," for instance, has less impact on a person's life than being able to "make a purchase," which in turn is less fulfilling than learning "how to shop." Help the person choose the "slice" of accomplishment that makes the most sense within the three-to-twelve month time frame.

continued from previous page

Shopping
- **Preparing shopping list**
- **Choosing food items**
- **Purchase exchanges**
- **Transportation**
- **Budgeting**
- **MONEY USAGE**

Cooking
- **Choosing meals**
- **Finding recipes**
- **Preparing ingredients**
- **Following recipes**
- **Measurement**
- **APPLIANCE USAGE**

Money Usage
- **Coin identification**
- **Bill identification**
- **Coin value**
- **Bill value**
- **Addition/subtraction**
- **Making change**

Appliance Usage
- **Microwave**
- **Oven**
- **Stove**
- **Toaster oven**
- **Blender**
- **Food processor**

With each reduction of a domain into further components, the learner becomes further removed from the original goal. In this example, "working on making change when using money" is far from the goal of "successfully living at home." The longer it will take to master each component skill related to the goal, the less likely it becomes that the individual will reach it unless adaptations, modifications, or assistance are provided (see next page).

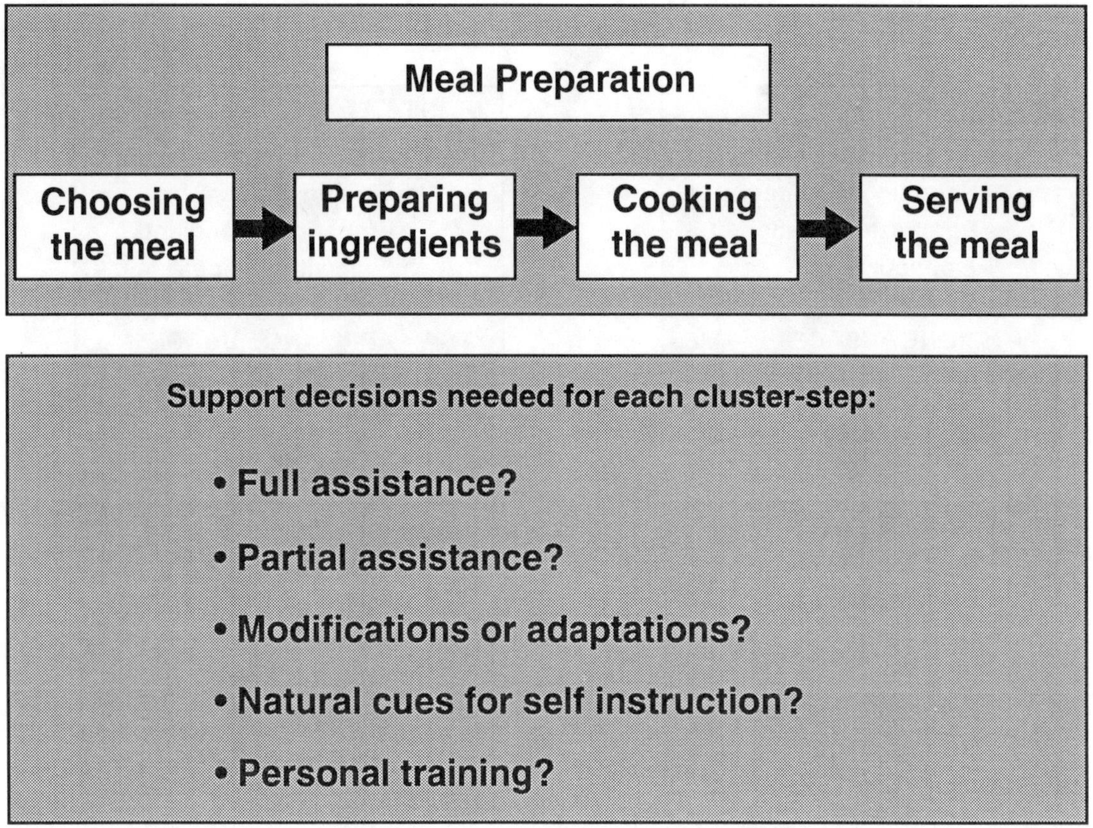

Many life dreams require certain sets of accomplishments. For example, to live independently, people need to be able to eat nutritiously. The entire process of meal preparation may be challenging to master for some persons. Rather than delaying or denying their preferences because of the time it might take to master a needed skill, it would be better to examine what aspects of that accomplishment could be learned by the person and what aspects need support. For example, what could be handled with changes to the oven, stove, microwave, or other tools of the kitchen? What things require direct assistance? How might that assistance be provided by the natural setting? What cues (picture recipe book, audiotape, etc.) could be provided so that the person could complete the task without assistance?

✦ Provide Help or Learn Just a Part of a Task?

Decisions should also be made about what to teach, what to adapt, or when to assist. These strategies should always be in the context of an individual's personal life and career goals and plans.

Some situations are better approached by providing assistance or modifications, rather than struggling for a long time to teach a skill that is difficult for someone to master (see illustration at left). This is a decision that must be made carefully and in coordination with the person and his or her family and service team.

Sometimes it may make sense for someone to learn only part of a complex task, rather than the whole thing. The concept that anyone is capable of learning some part of any task is called *partial participation* (Brown, et al., 1976).

This concept provides opportunities for persons to contribute and participate in community settings, even though they may not be able to do all parts of a particular task. The team must then explore how the remaining tasks will be completed. This may be accomplished through other supports or adaptations to the environment.

✦ Define Exactly What to Accomplish

Many people with disabilities learn best when taught precisely. Instead of leaving learning to chance, use precise, everyday language to clarify what needs to be mastered. For example:

- ✦ An *accomplishment* should be related through action verbs that describe observable behaviors by the *subject*.
- ✦ *Conditions* should define what needs to be present for the action to occur.
- ✦ *Criteria* for success should spell out when mastery occurs.
- ✦ *Measurement* standards should be chosen for their appropriateness to describe mastery.
- ✦ *Timelines* should define the expected date of mastery.

Sample Performance Objective

Because Susan wants to be more independent in her home, by 1/96 she will be able to plan, shop for, and prepare 5 different nutritious meals for 1 or 2 persons, using preferred recipes and a prepared budget.

Measurement:
Her level of independence will be indicated by: number of required cues to complete a task (planning, cooking, shopping); amount of time to complete cooking; quality of meal prepared as judged by Susan and others. Specific criteria for success for each meal will be developed.

Expected performance:
Less than 2 needed prompts per task; meal prep within recipe guidelines 3 of 4 times; quality of meal rated from 1 to 5, with 5 being excellent and 3 expected.

Notes:
Susan needs an adaptation to the stove, microwave, and oven to help her read the dials; she needs a modified dining schedule, sometimes with an invited guest so the size of the meal is appropriate. While these cooking skills will be helpful for her to learn, they are not prerequisites for her to move to her own apartment.

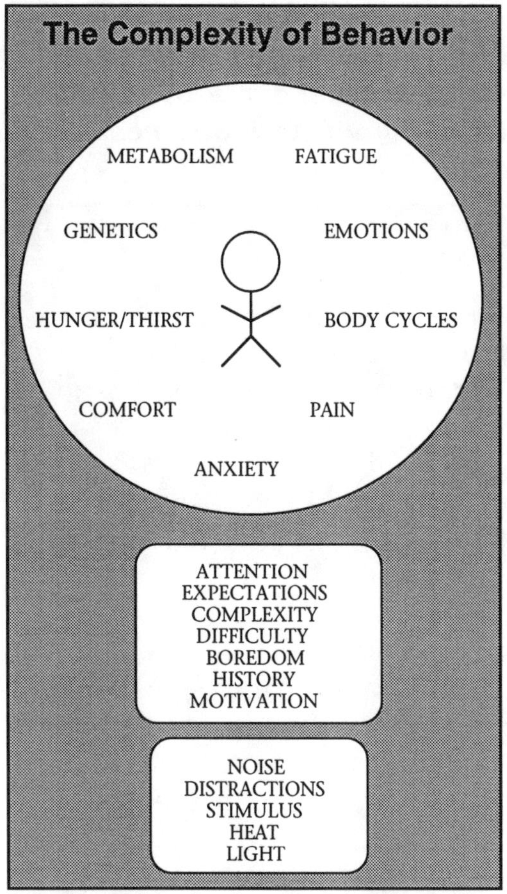

Behavior may be a function of very complex environmental and/or body processes. It is a mistake to assume a single cause of an action or to simplify the possibilities. Understanding behavior requires an exploration of an individual's life, health, desires, and situation, *and not just a program response.*

✦ Behavior

Some people have little experience or understanding of the norms of community life. As a result, they may act in socially unacceptable ways. To provide assistance, service providers will often help an individual determine and accomplish an objective to improve his or her behavior.

A behavioral objective such as this should never stand alone. It represents a technology to help someone realize an enhanced life goal. Listing an isolated behavioral "improvement" gives an out-of-context objective and accompanying behavioral program "a life of its own" that it does not deserve.

Instead, look at the behavior first as a possible *expression of communication* (Donnellan, et al., 1986). The true objective might be better realized by projecting changes in settings, activities, or relationships. Or perhaps further social experiences are needed for the individual to learn more about the implications of certain kinds of behavior (Lovett, 1985).

Behavior is very complex. There are many possible reasons why someone chooses to act in a certain way. Simply trying to change or "get rid of" a behavior without first attempting to understand it does a disservice to the individual.

Many times people are assumed incompetent to enter certain situations because of perceived inappropriate behaviors expressed in other human service environments. Closely examine and question these assumptions. It is important to guard an individual's reputation and safety, as well as the reputations and safety of those who will be present with an individual. But without being provided with an opportunity of community experience, persons will rarely achieve an arbitrary "readiness" standard in an over-structured, human service, behavior training program.

For example, if a person demonstrates certain self-stimulatory behaviors or aggressive/disruptive actions, it would be wise to provide support with behavioral technology. This assistance should be in the context of learning and achieving in settings and activities that are meaningful, integrated in the community, and provide value, prestige, and social connections.

The objective should focus on achievements in these domains, rather than the presence or absence of certain behaviors per se. The frequency of critical behaviors will be useful measures and indicators of the success towards the achievement objective, but are not the objective in and of themselves.

While it is beyond the scope of this publication to provide behavioral planning strategies, do use caution in writing objectives that focus on simply reducing inappropriate behaviors with no social context. Redirect efforts toward examining the quality of the individual's life and how positive changes can be achieved.

Sample Social Behavior Objective

Context:
Robin enjoys her job, but occasionally gets frustrated with a task and will yell loudly or throw things.

Objective: ***To keep a job she desires, Robin will learn the social expectations at work and understand the practical limitations that occur when she expresses her frustration through yelling and other disruptive actions. By March, 1996, she will be able to communicate, seek assistance, and wait for help in socially acceptable ways.***

Strategies:

- **When she needs assistance, help her learn to set her work aside and turn to other tasks available while she waits.**
- **Assist her to communicate her need for assistance through a signal, gesture, or other means.**
- **Provide encouragement when she is able to delay her desire for immediate help.**
- **Teach her how to request a break from work when she is feeling frustrated.**

Measurement:
Robin will increase her tolerance for frustration by being able to wait patiently for assistance for up to 10 minutes; by expressing her need for assistance with a regular tone of voice; by decreasing the number of times she expresses her frustration through yelling; and by being able to express any desire she has to make a change in her setting in socially acceptable ways.

Sample Employment Objectives

Pre-Statement Relating to Life Goal:

For Judy to have a meaningful career related to her interest in sports ...

For John to be able to earn the wages he desires for his own apartment ...

✦ Job Attainment (3-6 months)

Outcome: Employment at minimum specified hours, wages, etc.

John will be working at a clerical or office-related position for at least 20 hrs./wk. at minimum wage or better ...

Judy will be employed where her work will relate to her interests in ...

Strategies: Job tours, resume development, job experiences, interviews, job-seeking skills, career exploration.

✦ Job Performance (3-6 months)

Outcome: Production, efficiency, cooperation, wages, hours, self or employer satisfaction, stamina, etc.

Judy will increase her speed on 3 key work tasks identified by her employer to an acceptable level of productivity (See work strategies) ...

John will improve his wages to $175 per week through increased productivity and hours on his current job or with additional part-time work...

✦ Job Enhancement

Outcome: More responsibility, social relationships, participation, diversity, prestige, etc.

Judy will increase her responsibilities to include ...

John will become more included in his workplace as evidenced by his participation in the company softball team, sharing break-time snacks, and "after-hours" activities ...

✦ Job Advancement

Outcome: New title, more responsibility beyond original domains, position change, career change, increased wages, etc.

Judy will move into the clerical assistant position ...

John will begin to experience new career possibilities beyond maintenance positions in the areas of ... through part-time job experiences or ...

✦ Objectives Relating to Employment

With more and more individuals with disabilities seeking to enter the community workforce through supported employment, we should consider employment-specific objectives. Generally, there are four types of work goals:

- Job attainment
- Job performance
- Job enhancement
- Job advancement

Finding a job and learning a skill for that job are generally short-term objectives of only three to six months at most. If the objective is not achieved in that time, then the strategies used should be re-examined and changed.

✦ Identifying Natural Learning Opportunities

Before choosing learning priorities, assess how other persons are learning their skills in the setting in which the person will need to perform. Many community settings, particularly workplaces, have existing training programs and personnel who could provide instruction. The provider's role may be more of a consultant or planner rather than a direct trainer.

✦ Summary

Objectives are useful for breaking down complex achievement goals into manageable tasks that might take up to a year to master. They provide a process for measuring change and growth, documenting services, and providing feedback on what works and what does not.

Considerations in Developing Objectives

When objectives are used in helping to plan supports for an individual, the following should be considered:

1. **Choose high priority areas that will have an impact.**
2. **Select areas where realistic accomplishment is possible.**
3. **Include life goal context in stating objectives.**
4. **Pick the largest slice of accomplishment that represents the best scope of focus for the individual.**
5. **Help select measurements that reasonably match and measure the true content of the objective.**
6. **Be aware of the longevity of the plan. The people who implement the objectives are:**
    - **not likely to be at the team planning meeting,**
    - **will probably be new to the person,**
    - **will have to interpret the document with little history with the person or what is behind the objective.**
7. **Be aware of stigma and image when choosing objectives and strategies.**
8. **Use behavioral objectives in the context of a life goal, not in isolation.**

VI

Using Action Plans and Describing Routine Services

There are some individuals for whom a formal plan of objectives will not be appropriate. Their lives do not fit into a system developed around personal change and growth based on structured supports. They may be uncomfortable with a team of human service professionals or others helping to structure their lives.

For these individuals, an alternative to a detailed list of objectives is needed. One way to do this is to write an "action plan" consisting of a description of more informal supports and activities, based on the personal futures statement of the individual.

Another method is to provide and define a list of "routine services." This includes those supports expected on a routine and regular basis, their source, and how they will be reviewed.

What both have in common is a description of ongoing life patterns and their needed supports for a person, rather than a focus on personal development and attainment. For this reason, carefully consider utilizing either planning tool.

✦ Narrative, Flexible Format Defines Action Plans

An action plan uses a narrative and open format to describe the supports that an individual desires to maintain a certain lifestyle. Like other person-centered planning, it should occur in an informal setting such as at home or in a restaurant, where the individual can comfortably describe whatever types of support are needed.

Typically, the individual discusses what is desired with the person or persons who have the responsibility to help coordinate and negotiate the supports. This discussion takes the place of a "planning meeting."

Like all service plans, this plan's development and content are dictated by the individual, and revolve around the kinds of things needed for the person to live in a certain preferred manner, maintain health, work at a job, or access recreational or social pursuits.

These services might include transportation, budgeting advice, counseling, benefits planning, or other types

Elements of an Action Plan

- **Define areas in which support is needed and desired.**
- **Describe strategies for providing support.**
- **Note who is responsible for delivering each described support.**
- **Outline how the plan will be reviewed and agreements tracked.**
- **Note anything that might influence the course of the plan.**

Sample Action Plan Statements

Area: Transportation

Since Mary wishes to maintain her job of 7 years at the day care center, the agency will provide ongoing assistance as needed with transportation between work and home. This is expected to include funding for up to 5 taxi cab trips per month. No further support is required at the job site. Transportation assistance will be documented.

Area: Vacation

Mary would like to continue her routine of visiting her sister out of state for vacation each year. The agency will provide financial assistance of up to $500, as well as assist in planning, arranging transportation, lodging, and other budgeting as needed.

of assistance. These are described in relation to a person's situation.

In providing a narration of the action plan, include the context around each element of support. Describe why this type of support is desired by the individual in terms of the lifestyle he or she has chosen. For an example, see the box at left.

✦ Action Plan Should Be Authorized Prior to Development

Defining an action plan may be used in lieu of stating objectives. Check with the funding agency that has the overall responsibility for ISP development in your service region to see if an action plan will be acceptable for funding and accountability of services. Be certain it will meet any requirements the state or region may have for that particular person before you develop the plan.

To complete an action plan, follow the same types of processes described earlier in getting to know the person and his or her preferences, capabilities, attitudes, experiences, and situation. Act as a facilitator in drawing out the kinds of support that the person would find helpful in life.

Describe these areas in a brief narrative. Identify how the supports will be provided, who will provide them, when they will be provided, and how everyone will know if the individual is satisfied. Note any specific obstacles that you may need to handle. Finally, state how the person will check in with the individual coordinating service supports over the time between the plan's writing and its implementation.

✦ Routine Services

There are times when a great deal of the services to be provided to an individual are ongoing and routine in nature, as opposed to growth-related services which support the attainment of new skills or lifestyles. When a team decides that it is appropriate, these routine services can be noted as part of an individual's plan.

Various regions of a state may have different forms or lists of services that are expected from providers of particular services. These lists are usually typical life services for home, community, or employment, such as:

Personal Care
- obtaining/preparing medications
- bathing/showering
- toothbrushing/dental care
- toileting skills
- menstrual needs
- hair care
- nail care
- dressing appropriately
- laundry skills

Home Care
- household chores (vacuuming, dusting, mopping, sweeping, dish washing, room cleaning, etc.)
- household safety procedures
- fire and emergency evacuation procedures
- developing daily routines

Financial Assistance
- budgeting to meet fixed and regular expenses, allowing for personal spending
- paying bills
- purchase of medications, clothing, household items, groceries, personal items
- feedback on priorities of purchases
- retaining receipts and check stubs for reporting to IRS and SSI as appropriate
- advice on means of obtaining major purchases through reviewing resources available and savings
- assistance if conflict with bills arises

Nutrition Assistance
- advice on menu planning
- grocery list
- proper storage of food items
- meal prep as needed
- teaching meal prep skills desired by individual

Community-Based Skills
- personal and emergency telephone use
- street safety
- community public transportation
- shopping
- banking
- recreational/leisure activities

Sample Routine Service List

- **Safety and evacuation**
- **Financial assistance**
- **Shopping/purchasing**
- **Benefits management**
- **Meals and nutrition**
- **Accessing community services**
- **Transportation**
- **Use of telephone**
- **Personal care**
- **Domestic care**
- **Health care**
- **Special therapies**
- **Dental care**
- **Recreational support**
- **Specialized equipment**
- **Church attendance**

Besides listing the routine services to be provided as above, the service plan should also specify the frequency of service supports, describe the service for the individual, the source of the support, and how the service will be periodically reviewed.

Developing Relationships:
• identifying activities/groups of interest
• attending get-togethers of friends/ relatives/groups
• proactive effort in connecting the individual with other community members

✦ Summary

Action plans are useful alternatives to more data-oriented plans. They can be developed instead of using formal objectives for those persons who do not require more structured services.

Check first with someone who has the capability of authorizing an action plan for a particular individual before you begin to develop it.

Sometimes a list of straightforward services or supports that are routine in nature is all the individual wishes or requires. A list of these routine services, along with their frequency and source, may be included in the ISP.

VII

Putting It Together: Facilitation and Follow-Up

As described in the previous pages, developing a service plan for a person with a disability is far more than simply attending a meeting to write a few objectives. Much preparation and investment of knowledge and time needs to be done by all the team members.

✦ Who Composes a Planning Team?

There is no fixed membership for a team other than the individual who needs support and the person responsible for coordinating it. Other participants can range from friends, family, guardians, and service providers to co-workers and professional consultants.

The key elements are interest, connection, and respect for the person for whom the planning is intended. The individual himself or herself should be the source of generating invitations to others to participate. This is his or her meeting, not the service coordinator's or the program's.

In fact, some people may prefer to plan without a group meeting. You can respect this preference by gathering information and ideas with people the person identifies one at a time.

✦ How Often Should a Team Meet?

Teams are required to meet at least annually to update service plans, evolve new plans, and make revisions. When people's lives and needs change more frequently, the team should come together more often. For example, if the individual loses a job or starts a new one, or if the person is changing where they live or with whom they live, a meeting might be considered.

Also, if the person is facing a challenging situation or trying to reach an accomplishment, the team may wish to regularly gather for mini-sessions and updates, much as the circles of support concept recommends.

Any member of the team may seek out the individual with a disability and his or her service coordinator to suggest a meeting of the full team or a partial grouping of the team. This can be done as often as needed.

> **"The role of the facilitator is to elicit participation of all team members in the collective design of an integrated ... community life."**
>
> Terri Vandercook
> Jennifer York

Roles of the Facilitator

- Monitor group process
- Help the focus person stay the center of planning
- Keep the group on-task
- Seek equal participation
- Help direct discussion and seek information
- Document the proceedings and outcomes
- Review action steps
- Acknowledge commitments and responsibilities of team members

✦ Pre-Meeting Preparation

The team facilitator should help the individual for whom the planning is intended to provide invitations in advance. The person's own words on personalized notecards can work very well.

Input should be sought from those who are unable to attend. The meeting facilitator should ask participants to spend time thinking about how they can help the planning process.

Deciding where to hold the meeting is another important factor. Help the person to chose a place where everyone can attend, be comfortable, feel free to speak, and be productive.

Coffee and snacks often help add informality and comfort. It's also helpful to have large newsprint paper and a marker ready so that all participants will be able to see it. This allows ideas to be recorded visually so that all may feel a sense of accomplishment as the process builds.

✦ Establish Trust

The facilitator needs to establish an atmosphere of trust where risk-taking is allowed and valued. This requires an investment of time for relationship building, respectful exchanges, social support for contributions, and a light touch of humor when appropriate.

As team participants grow more comfortable with their own participation and the various roles of other people in the group, they will feel more secure in speaking up.

Many times professionals use jargon that sounds like an unknown language to community or family members. This can stifle trust, creativity and communication.

If necessary, the facilitator should translate the opinions of professionals into words everyone will understand. This will have the added benefit of keeping the process grounded in everyday reality.

✦ How Should Meetings Be Conducted?

Since quality of life is different for each person, each team process should be unique. This does not mean an unplanned gathering where "anything goes." Time is an important resource. Purposeful meetings should have clear desired outcomes. There should be a respect of the individual's wishes as the center of planning. Usually the facilitator, after making sure each person is comfortable, welcomes everyone, thanks them for coming, and asks for introductions.

From there, the process will vary according to the characteristics of the team. It may be useful to start the meeting with a brief description of the current situation and what the individual hopes to accomplish with the meeting. Although this can be done by anyone or by everyone, it is best done by the focus person if possible. It should be concise, last less than a few minutes, and set the stage for the rest of the meeting.

If previous meetings already have developed useful planning and information, don't waste time redoing what has already been done. Review these outcomes in terms of today's changing needs. This may provide perspective and a planning starting point. It may also help illustrate what has been tried, what seems to help, and what does not seem to work. There may be a review of previous goals, successes, and challenges.

Once this is accomplished, the participants get down to business using whatever process is most effective for that group. There may be brainstorming of next steps, or a discussion of whatever is of highest priority. Again, there are no fixed formulas to review and develop a plan of service to assist someone to achieve a sought-after quality of life.

There are, however, effective meetings and time-wasting ones, respectful and degrading meetings, creative ones and rigid ones. More effective and purposeful team gatherings support the approaches to planning stated at right.

Positive Approaches to Planning Personal Futures

- **The individual's wishes are the center of planning.**
- **Team members represent a mix of community members, friends, and professionals.**
- **All team members contribute.**
- **Creativity is used in building services.**
- **Supports and services are developed around the person instead of placing the person into fixed services.**
- **Approaches and responses remain flexible.**
- **Expectations are high but attainable.**

Yielding to others' opinions just to avoid a conflict is counterproductive. Team members should be flexible and open to new ideas, but be able to refuse suggestions that they consider to be unsound.

✦ Facilitation and Team Dynamics

To accomplish their purpose, teams must be conducted skillfully. A facilitator should ensure that discussion flows respectfully around a person's capacities rather than deficits. People should attend the meeting with their knowledge of the person, along with ideas for how assistance may be provided. This is far different than attending a meeting with a fixed agenda, pre-written objectives, or a pre-developed program.

Meetings should not be too long or over-focused on a single issue. The facilitator must be able to keep discussion moving without shutting down participants, so that the person's full life desires can be assisted.

When people come together to form a group, interactions get more complex. Emotions can develop, based on the feelings people have about how they stand within the group.

These emotions can cloud judgements, cause people to hold back or exaggerate their participation, or make people focus on unimportant issues for far too much time. Thus, every group must invest in understanding how to build a working team where the members support each other.

✦ Building Consensus

Not everyone will always agree on the best way to prioritize a needed service or how to deliver it. It is up to the facilitator to try to build a consensus of direction. The facilitator should do this by taking cues from the individual needing support (and family/guardians), either from previous discussions or opinions expressed at the meeting.

Differences of opinion are not necessarily bad. They often can lead to a more diverse and creative array of possible support. If a team can be open to wide ranging ideas, a fuller exploration of resources may be possible.

To keep ideas flowing, the facilitator should be in tune with the group process. An effective facilitator will redirect dominating team members, ask quiet team members for their opinions and thoughts, and help translate any jargon from professionals.

Many times, community members or family members are intimidated by human service professionals. The facilitator should demystify the opinions of professionals, with all due respect, as partners in a process with a useful perspective to offer.

If the discussion seems to be heading in no direction or toward a dead-end, put the process on hold and move to another topic. Finally, if the meeting is getting bogged down in a conflict or difference of opinion, the facilitator may wish to postpone the process (or the particular topic of dispute) until more facts can be explored.

Outcomes of Effective Service Plans

- **There is a balanced description of strengths, interests, and needs.**
- **Services flow from personal preferences.**
- **Future visions are based on personalized dreams and goals.**
- **Services are integrated among disciplines in context to life goals.**
- **Circles of relationships evolve as a result of planning.**

Features to Avoid in Service Plans

- **Use of jargon**
- **Focus on needs based on deficits**
- **Overuse of labels and diagnosis**
- **Splintered interdisciplinary teams**
- **Goals based only on what programs offer**
- **Formal and rigid process that flows from providers**
- **Restrictive documents left behind**
- **Product does not describe the real person**
- **Overemphasis on objectivity and trivial measures**
- **"Fix the person" attitude**
- **Low expectations**

"There are many times ... we have experienced a phenomenon which can be described by the blowing out of our candle. We are tired, discouraged, frustrated, ready to give up. Here is where the gifts and capacities of each in a circle of support come to bear. We have found there is always someone ready to share his or her candle to light another's again. Strength is renewed on 'together' to the next part of the journey."

Pat Beeman,
George Ducharme,
Beth Mount

✦ Follow-Up

Implementing the services described in the plan is the second biggest challenge after developing the service plan itself. This is the real beginning of services, not the end of team planning.

Too many traditional human service programs invest time in writing a plan that is never reviewed or thought of again until a year later when it is the perceived time to rewrite the plan. This is then done with no thought or perspective from the previous year's success or disappointments.

Once some direction and strategies have been developed, there should be follow-up to review approaches, efforts, resources, personnel, community changes, and life changes. Service providers may need the guidance of family members or professional specialists to meet the individual's objectives. There should be a lot of communication, discussion, and feedback on how services are developing between team members at this time.

✦ Plans Have a Useful Life, but Must Evolve with the Person

People's needs evolve unevenly, not in nice annual boxes of time. When major change occurs, seek out the guidance of the individual and his or her team members in revising the planned service strategies. Just because an objective is written down doesn't mean it has a life of its own. When circumstances change, the plan must change to reflect those changes.

✦ Negotiating Change with Service Systems

The following thoughts are useful to consider when a planning team or facilitator reaches an impasse with a bureaucracy about services or supports for an individual (Des Jardins, 1980).

1. Do not feel guilty, insignificant, or apologetic when asking for services.
2. Do not beg for what a person is entitled to by law.
3. Do not be overly patient. Time needed will expand to time allowed.

4. Do not be hostile. Provide empathy and support for difficult issues, yet remain firm.
5. Offer support as an ally when resources are needed to fulfill a commitment.
6. Do not let issues accelerate to become a "system problem." Stay focused on the individual.
7. Be clear, concise, and articulate about your expectations.
8. Always put in writing negotiations and understandings made.
9. Do not let yourself be buried with overwhelming excuses or rationalizations. They can continue indefinitely.
10. Don't let agencies pass the buck.

✦ Summary

The development of an ISP requires a prepared approach that is open, centers around the person's skills, interests, and capacities, and utilizes the planning tools provided in this manual. Once the team gathers to actually document the plan, effective facilitation is needed to keep the team creative and to build consensus. The documentation of the plan is really the beginning of services and not the end of the team. Follow-up is needed so that team members communicate and remain true to the expressed wishes of the individual in his or her pursuit of a quality life.

References

Beeman, Pat, Ducharme, George, and Mount, Beth (1989). *One Candle Power: Building Bridges into Community Life for People with Disabilities*. Manchester, CT: Communitas, Inc.

Brown, Lou, Nietupski, John, and Hamre-Nietupski, S. (1976). The Criterion of Ultimate Functioning. In M.A. Thomas (Ed.), *Hey, Don't Forget about Me!*Reston, VA: Council for Exceptional Children.

Callahan, Michael (1991). The Role of Evaluation: Traditional Uses and Emerging Practices. *Systematic Instruction for Supported Employment*. Mark Gold and Associates.

Des Jardins, Charlotte (1980). *How to Organize an Effective Parent/Advocacy Group and Move Bureaucracies*. Chicago: Coordinating Council for Handicapped Children.

DiLeo, Dale (1990; 1993). *Enhancing the Lives of Adults with Disabilities*. St. Augustine, FL: Training Resource Network.

Donnellan, Anne, Mirenda, Pat, Mesaros, R. and Fassbender, L. (1986). Analyzing the Communicative Function of Aberrant Behavior. *Journal of The Association for Persons with Severe Handicaps, 9*.

Knoll, J. and Ford, Allison. (1987). Beyond Caregiving: A Reconceptualization of the Role of the Residential Service Provider. In Taylor, Steve, Biklen, Doug, and Knoll, James. (Eds.), *Community Integration for People with Severe Disabilities*. Teacher's College, Columbia University, NY: Teacher's College Press.

Forest, Marsha, and Snow, Judith (1987). *The MAPS PROCESS*. Frontier College, Toronto.

Lovett, Herb (1985). *Cognitive Counseling and Persons with Special Needs*. New York: Praeger Publishers.

McKnight, John (1988). Associational Map. *The Future of Low-Income Neighborhoods and the People Who Reside There*. Center for Urban Affairs and Policy Research, Northwestern University.

McKnight, John (1988). *Do No Harm: A Policymaker's Guide to Evaluating Human Services and Their Alternatives*. Center for Urban Affairs and Policy Research, Northwestern University.

McKnight, John (1989). *Beyond Community Services*. Center for Urban Affairs and Policy Research, Northwestern University.

Mount, Beth (1987). *Personal Futures Planning: Finding Directions for Change*. Unpublished dissertation, University of GA.

Mount, Beth, Beeman, Pat and Ducharme, George (1988). *What Are We Learning about Circles of Support: A Collection of Tools, Ideas, and Reflections on Building and Facilitating Circles of Support*. Manchester, CT: Communitas, Inc.

Mount, Beth, Beeman, Pat and Ducharme, George (1988). *What Are We Learning about Bridge-Building? A Summary of a Dialogue between People Seeking to Build Community for People with Disabilities*. Manchester, CT: Communitas, Inc.

O'Brien, John and Lovett, Herbert (1992). *Finding a Way Toward Everyday Lives: The Contribution of Person Centered Planning*. Harrisburg, PA: Pennsylvania Office of Mental Retardation.

O'Brien, John and Lyle, Connie (1987). *Design for Accomplishment*. Lithonia, GA: Responsive Systems Associates.

O'Brien, John (1987). A Guide to Lifestyle Planning. *A Comprehensive Guide to the Activities Catalog*. Baltimore: Paul H. Brookes Publishing Co.

O'Brien, J. (1980). The Principle of Normalization: A Foundation for Effective Services. In Gardener, J.F., Long, L., Nichols, R., & Iagulli, D. (Eds.), *Program Issues in Developmental Disabilities*. Baltimore: Paul H. Brookes Publishing Co.

Perske, Robert (1988). *Circles of Friends*. Nashville, TN: Abingdon Press.

Perske, Robert (1980). *New Life in the Neighborhood*. Nashville, TN: Abingdon Press.

Snow, Judith, and Forest, Marsha (1986). *Support Circles - Building a Vision*, Roehr Institute.

Turnbull, Ann and Turnbull, Rud (1993). *Group Action Planning: Families, Friends, and Professionals*. University of KS: Beach Center on Families and Disability.

Vandercook, Terri, and York, Jennifer (1988). Integrated Education: MAPS to Get You There. Minnesota *UAP IMPACT*, Vol 1 (2), Winter.

Wolfensberger, W. (1972). *Normalization in Human Services*. Toronto: National Institute on Mental Retardation.

Wolfensberger, W. (1983). Social Role Valorization: A Proposed New Term for the Principle of Normalization. *Mental Retardation, 21*, 234-239.